Effective Ways to Lose Weight without Starving

Natural Weight Loss Methods Outlined

By: Angela Turner

9781630225872

I0455926

TABLE OF CONTENTS

PUBLISHERS NOTES

Speedy Publishing LLC

40 E. Main St., #1156

Newark, DE 19711

www.speedypublishing.co

Cover Artwork: 24 Hr. Designs Ltd.

Editing: Speedy Publishing LLC

Book design: Speedy Publishing LLC

ISBN: 9781630225872

This is a reprint book.

DISCLAIMER

This publication is intended to provide helpful and informative material. It is not intended to diagnose, treat, cure, or prevent any health problem or condition, nor is intended to replace the advice of a physician. No action should be taken solely on the contents of this book. Always consult your physician or qualified health-care professional on any matters regarding your health and before adopting any suggestions in this book or drawing inferences from it.

The author and publisher specifically disclaim all responsibility for any liability, loss or risk, personal or otherwise, which is incurred as a consequence, directly or indirectly, from the use or application of any contents of this book.

Any and all product names referenced within this book are the trademarks of their respective owners. None of these owners have sponsored, authorized, endorsed, or approved this book.

Always read all information provided by the manufacturers' product labels before using their products. The author and publisher are not responsible for claims made by manufacturers.

DEDICATION

For Janice, Christine and Becky - Don't you miss our days of gaining and losing weight from our fad diets?

INTRODUCTION

Are you carrying a little extra weight around the middle? Maybe you've got more than just a little weight problem – maybe it's a rather large one and you need to get rid of the fat for health reasons. Rest assured that you're not alone!

Obesity in America is at an all-time high. One of out of every three Americans is obese – a number that has doubled in just ten years. This epidemic is growing out of control in other countries as well as fast food franchises open in China, Japan, Germany, and other industrialized nations. When you are overweight, it's a serious issue. Carrying extra weight can make you more susceptible to heart problems, diabetes, stroke, and various types of cancer. It can also affect your body image as well thus causing problems with your self-esteem.

You deserve to be healthier and take off some of that weight that is making you unhealthy. But what if you're like me and love food so you hate the idea of having to eat rice cakes and alfalfa sprouts or starving yourself just to help the weight come off. We have good news for you! You don't have to starve yourself to lose weight!

Many people associate weight loss with being hungry all the time. They're afraid to start a weight loss plan because they want to avoid the frustrations of hunger. And yes, a lot of times for many people they think it's better to be overweight than to starve. I'm no exception. I really like to eat, so there's no way I would be constantly hungry for the sake being thin. What kind of life is it if you're always feeling hungry?

Our natural instinct tells us to eat when we are hungry. Hunger is a signal telling the body that it needs to eat. It is also a signal to the body that it is in danger, that it needs food now. Our self-preservation instinct makes us scarf down everything in sight in response to feelings of starvation.

Our body doesn't care that we live in the modern world where food is plentiful. It acts the same as it would if we were living in a wild, having to hunt for our food. And it is not wise to go against the instinct that is designed to protect us from starvation death.

So, get ready for a surprise: you do not have to be hungry in order to lose weight. On the contrary, eating regular meals and keeping yourself full is what will actually help you stick to your healthy eating plan and reach your goals. Keeping your hunger in check will help you avoid overeating. It will also prevent you from feeling miserable, frustrated and out of control.

Diet and weight loss is big business these days. It seems you're always seeing and hearing ads for weight loss products that promise amazing results. Some of them have their own meal plans, some are just small little pills that purport to burn fat, and others ask you to cut certain foods out of your diet in order to adjust the body's metabolism. There are many, many people out there who have amazing success using these programs. Kirstie Alley's looking great these days with Jenny Craig, and there's no denying that Anna Nicole Smith has regained her image as a sex symbol with Trim Spa.

The downside to these companies and diet plans is that they can often be expensive. The pills you take for weight loss can contain dangerous chemicals or have a large amount of caffeine that make you jittery and feel out of control. The positives are that they are easy to follow and provide you with support when you have questions or just need a positive uplift on the way to your goal weight. If you want to join these programs, that's wonderful! But know that everything they offer you can be done all on your own.

Angela Turner

You can prepare the meals that Jenny Craig offers, you can gain the same effect that those fat burning pills give, you can be in control of your own weight loss program – and you don't have to starve to do it! Inside the pages of this book, we'll give you all kinds of tips and tricks toward successful weight loss. We'll examine some common weight loss myths and even give you some great recipes to try while you are on this journey. It won't be easy and you'll have to maintain your willpower to be successful, but losing weight without starving yourself is a goal YOU CAN achieve.

CHAPTER 1- WHY ARE WE SO OVERWEIGHT?

Obesity is the leading cause of death and triggers the onset of many disease like diabetes.

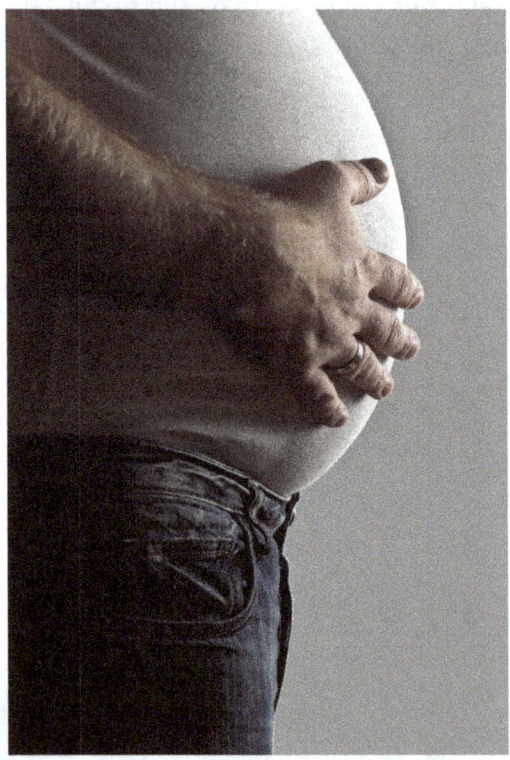

I suppose the easiest answer is fast food, but the problem extends out to so much more. Yes, the prevalence of fast food restaurants certainly doesn't help. As Morgan Spurlock showed us with painful reality in his movie, "Super Size Me", fast food menus offer us a heaping helping of fat, cholesterol, and calories. I highly recommend watching this movie if you find yourself addicted to McDonald's – you could very well change your mind after you see it! At any rate, many of these restaurants are now offering health-conscious choices including salads, potatoes instead of French fries, yogurt, and grilled meats instead of fried meats. So with these items now included on their menu, why aren't we losing weight? The answer lies within our choices. Those choices extend to home life as well. Many people live horridly busy lifestyles, and they more often than not opt for pre-packaged foods that contain high amounts of salt, fat, and other unhealthy components that contribute toward weight gain. We tend to maintain a mostly sedentary lifestyle choosing to watch a favorite television program after dinner rather than going out for a walk like they used to do decades ago. This type of life style unfortunately is being learned by our children as well. When I was young, we couldn't wait to get through dinner so we could go outside and play a game of kick the can as the sun went down. We rode our bikes everywhere and only watched television when "The Brady Bunch" or "The Partridge Family" was on. Hey, we had our priorities!

Today, you're more likely to find kids on the computer or in front of the TV with a video game controller in their hands. Kids know more about the story line on Desperate Housewives than many of their housewife mothers. They can tell you about all of the new products being offered through commercials they see in between their programs. In fact, the average child these days will watch more than 15 hours of television each and every week. Now, we're not saying television is BAD. In fact, some programs can be beneficial and even helpful in making kids smarter. What we're saying is that kids need to get outside more instead of sitting in front of the TV eating Cheetos and drinking sugar rich soda.

The statistics are showing this to be true. Fifteen percent of all children and teens are overweight - a number that has tripled since a previous study done in 1980. Some people blame their excessive weight gain on slow metabolisms. In some cases, this might actually be true. However, the Center for Disease Control (CDC) has confirmed what no one really wants to face: we're overweight because we simply eat too much of the wrong foods.

Losing weight is actually quite simple – eat less, exercise more. But we're resistant to that message. Mainly, it's because we're looking for a quick fix – an easy, painless way to drop pounds without sacrifice. After all, losing weight just CAN'T be that easy, now can it? No, it isn't. You have to consider portion control, food choice, exercise, how much exercise, what kind of exercise, etc. But worrying about all of the specifics will do you little good. You need to get the big picture in mind first before worrying about the specifics.

What you want to do is lose those extra pounds. And there are many, many ways to go about that. But before you wait around for the next miracle diet, try some of the tried and true methods we'll show you. It's not as monumental as you think it is!

CHAPTER 2- METABOLISM AND YOUR WEIGHT

Persons with a slower metabolism tend to gain weight much more quickly than someone with a fast metabolism.

You likely know your metabolism is linked to your weight. But do you know how?

Common belief holds that a slim person's metabolism is high and an overweight person's metabolism is low. But this isn't usually the case. Metabolism alone doesn't determine your weight.

Rather, weight is dependent on the balance of calories consumed versus calories burned. Take in more calories than your body needs, and you gain weight. Take in less and you lose weight. Metabolism, then, is the engine that burns these calories and is the scale that regulates your energy needs.

Stated simply, metabolism is the process by which your body converts food into energy. During this biochemical process, calories — from carbohydrates, fats and proteins —are combined with oxygen to release the energy your body needs to function.

The number of calories your body burns each day is called your total energy expenditure. The following three factors make up your total energy expenditure:

- Basic needs. Even when your body is at rest, it requires energy for the basics, such as fuel for organs, breathing, circulating blood, adjusting hormone levels, plus growing and repairing cells.

Calories expended to cover these basic functions are your basal metabolic rate.

- Typically, a person's basal metabolic rate is the largest portion of energy use, representing two-thirds to three-quarters of the calories used each day. Energy needs for these basic functions stay fairly consistent and aren't easily changed.
- Food processing. Digesting, absorbing, transporting and storing the food you consume also takes calories. This accounts for about 10 percent of the calories used each day. For the most part, your body's energy requirement to process food stays relatively steady and isn't easily changed.
- Physical activity. Physical activity — such as playing tennis, walking to the store, chasing after the dog and any other movement — accounts for the remainder of calories used. You control the number of calories burned depending on the frequency, duration and intensity of your activities.

It may seem logical to think that significant weight gain or being overweight is related to a low metabolism or possibly even a condition such as under-active thyroid gland (hypothyroidism). In reality, it's very uncommon for excess weight to be related to a low metabolism. And most people who are overweight don't have an underlying condition, such as hypothyroidism. However, a medical evaluation can determine whether a medical condition could be influencing your weight.

Weight gain is more likely due to an energy imbalance — consuming more calories than your body burns. To lose weight, then, you need to create an energy deficit by eating fewer calories, increasing the number of calories you burn through physical activity, or preferably both. If you and everyone else were physically and functionally identical, it would be easy to determine the standard energy needs. But many factors influence calorie requirements, including body size and composition, age, and sex.

To function properly, a bigger body mass requires more energy (more calories) than does a smaller body mass. Also, muscle burns more calories than fat does. So the more muscle you have in relation to fat, the higher your basal metabolic rate.

As you get older, the amount of muscle tends to decrease and fat accounts for more of your weight. Metabolism also slows naturally with age. Together these changes reduce your calorie needs. Men usually have less body fat and more muscle than do women of the same age and weight. This is why men generally have a higher basal metabolic rate and burn more calories than women do.

Your ability to change your basal metabolism is limited. However, you can increase daily exercise and activity to build muscle tissue and burn more calories. Your metabolism influences your energy needs, but it's your food intake and physical activity that ultimately determine your weight.

Losing weight, like any task you undertake, requires that you have dedication and motivation to succeed. This means you need to get your head in the right place.

CHAPTER 3- GETTING INTO THE RIGHT MINDSET

Without the right attitude, an individual will never lose weight or achieve anything else.

Believe it or not, there is a psychological factor that comes into play when you're trying to lose weight. We like to compare it to the "rah rah" factor that you sometimes need to succeed in sports.

Look at your weight loss as your own personal sporting event. Just as you need to know the rules of the game as well as the basics of performing that game in sports, you also need the right information in your diet to make it effective.

When you have all the tools you need, you can become an excellent performer in almost anything you try in life. One of these tools is the right frame of mind. The right frame of mind will give you motivation, commitment, and the skills you need to overcome the obstacles that you might face along with temptations and distractions. Think this sounds a little too "new age" for you? Think again! When you have the right psychology during your weight loss journey, you will make your weight loss fun, easier, more exciting, and be able to develop changes towards a healthier lifestyle that will stay with you forever. Your mindset controls your behavior, actions, and thoughts. As people grow, they develop habits and associations that govern their life. Most of these habits are controlled by our sub-conscious and we are generally unaware of them. However, your subconscious could also sabotage your efforts – also while you unaware of them. This can be detrimental to your weight loss attempts. The right mindset entails using various techniques and strategies to control your behavior by monitoring your thoughts and actions. When you obtain this mindset, you will be better equipped to replace the old habits and associations that formed your thinking in the first place with new and more positive habits that will enable you to lost weight and be happier while you do so! Developing the correct mindset doesn't occur overnight. It take a little bit of effort, but in the end, it is well worth the time you'll spend doing so. You will have to regularly monitor your progress and behavior. Sometimes it will be easy – at other times, it won't. The good news is that there are some easy ways to begin to put yourself into the right mindset.

1. Write your goals down – tell yourself what weight you want to get to. While you're at it, write down any other personal goals you might have as far as your life in general. Since you're undertaking something as huge as losing your extra weight, you may as well also focus your efforts on improving other aspects of your life while you have the motivation and drive.

2. Be specific about what those goals are. When you generalize your goals, you are trivializing them. Your goals ARE IMPORTANT. Make them important!

3. Assign yourself a deadline. You want to lose weight.

4. You want to do it by Christmas, or your wedding, or the next class reunion. When you assign a deadline, you give yourself a goal to work for, and like we said, your goals ARE IMPORTANT!

5. Make those goals measurable and achievable. Don't think TOO big or try to undertake more than what you are capable of. If you need to lose 100 pounds, don't expect to do it in a few weeks. Give yourself enough time to do so in a healthy manner. You could also try to break the goals down into

easier increments. Tell yourself that you will lose 10 pounds over the next month. Then tell yourself the same thing the next month. Eventually, you'll reach that goal and feel the satisfaction of being lighter than you were before.

6. Focus on those goals every day. Post them on your refrigerator. Write them in your date book. Put a reminder on the visor of your car. When you focus on your goals, you will keep them in mind all the time and when they are first and foremost in your mind, you will be well on the way toward achieving them.

7. Be committed to those goals – at all costs. There's a reason why you want to achieve those goals. When you are committed, those goals become the focus of your mind and they will be much easier to realize. The battle with our metabolism as we age can't be denied. Our metabolism, which transforms our food into energy, slows down with each passing year. If we don't adjust our eating habits and our exercise to compensate, we slowly add additional pounds. We may feel betrayed, but the reality is we're going to have to change some habits in order to maintain our weight.

If you take things one step at a time, there are basic steps that can be adopted. Stop telling yourself, "I just can't do it." You can coax yourself into a new habit of healthy eating.

Developing a psychology towards weight loss will help you achieve you goals and realize success. Aim high, push yourself to become the type of person you want to be and live the life that you want and deserve. We are not given the power of dreams without the

power and ability to achieve those dreams. It's time to start —
RIGHT NOW!

CHAPTER 4- WHAT ABOUT THOSE DIET COMPANIES AND FAD DIETS?

Not all advertised diets are actually beneficial. A lot of them force persons to starve for a period of time and of course weight is lost but when the diet is over, the weight is quickly regained.

We'll start out here by saying unequivocally that we think that many of these companies such as Jenny Craig and Weight Watchers have their definite positive aspects. They give people a way to lose weight in a healthy manner by providing foods you can eat that will meet recommended caloric intakes. They also give support and advice along the way as you lose weight.

Their downfall is that they can be quite expensive to join when you factor in the cost of membership along with the food. Many of these companies require you to buy their own pre-packaged food for all meals, and that can get quite costly. They are a good option for those of you who can well afford their plans and can stick to them. There are also many, many fad diets that have popped up over the years that promise rapid weight loss as long as you stick to their recommendations. Some of these fad diets, however, can be dangerous, and they should be carefully evaluated before they are undertaken. One such diet is the low carb option such as the Atkins Diet Plan. While many people have been able to lose weight using this plan, others have reported some serious health concerns about this.

Low carb diets can help you lose weight quickly, but keeping that weight off becomes much more difficult once the diet isn't followed faithfully. Because of the requirements of the diet – high protein, no "white foods", etc. – you will be eating foods that are generally high in fat which can raise cholesterol levels.

Some of the claims made by people who advocate low carb diets just don't hold up. Because of the nature of the diet plan, you will lose weight quickly by cutting out carbs, but you won't be able to keep it off once you re-introduce those carbohydrates back into your eating plan. In fact, the longer you are on a low carb diet, the more quickly you will re-gain your old weight.

Carbohydrates provide a way for your body to convert food into energy. By keeping them out of your diet, you'll notice a lowering of your energy level, and your muscles will lose their tone becoming softer and flattening out. Also consider that these types of diets recommend that you eat a lot of protein which would be mostly meats and fish. Many of these foods are high in fat. Eating a lot of fat can contribute to health problems like heart disease, high blood pressure, and some cancers.

Yes, low carb diets can help you lose weight quickly, but know completely what you're getting into before you start. A good diet plan will balance out all the things your body needs to operate efficiently in terms of food and the benefits of those foods.

You may also be considering one of the many "fat burner" pills out there advertised everywhere. It seems like everyone time I turn on the television, I see a commercial showing people who've lost 100 pounds in just two weeks and now they can parade around in swimsuits on national TV – all with the help of the amazing diet pill they'd been taking.

Some people have great luck losing weight by taking these pills, but those pills do come with risks attached to them. These pills are not required to be tested by the Food and Drug Administration (FDA) before they are released to the public.

On the upside, if the drug is found to be dangerous, the FDA will work quickly to make sure it is banned from future sales. This happened in 2003 when the FDA banned products that contained ephedrine after it was found to be at least partly responsible for the death of a prominent athlete. These pills work in different ways. Many are appetite suppressants containing phenylpropanoline or caffeine. Some claim to increase your metabolism thus increasing the body's ability to burn fat while at the same time causing you to feel less hungry. Other pills say they can block the body's ability to absorb fat or help you lose weight by removing fluids from the body. These pills contain a diuretic or laxative.

It's very important for you to consult with your doctor before you start taking any kind of diet pills – even the ones that claim to be all-natural. This is especially true if you have a medical condition. Taking these pills could interact with medication you are already taking or it could aggravate a previous condition such as anxiety disorders. Diet pills can be addictive, so take caution when beginning their regimen. Follow the directions for dosages exactly and be aware of any possible side effects. If you experience any of the following symptoms while taking diet pills, stop taking them immediately and consult with your physician:

- Anxiety or nervousness

- Irritability

- Insomnia, restlessness, or hyperactivity

- High blood pressure

- Tightening in the chest

- Heart palpitations

- Fever

- Dry mouth

- Excessive headaches

- Dizziness

- Blurred Vision

- Profuse sweating

- Menstrual cycle or sex drive disturbances

Because diet pills can be purchased over the counter, it is up to each individual person to use them correctly. Some people stupidly take more than the recommended dosage in hopes that it will speed up the weight loss, but this is very dangerous! You can overdose on diet pills which can cause tremors, breathing problems, convulsions, renal failure or heart attack.

If you want to take diet pills, that is certainly one way for you to try and lose weight. Just do so cautiously and follow the manufacturer's instructions exactly in order to keep yourself safe. Even if you do take diet pills, you will still have to make modifications to your diet and introduce exercise in order to lose weight. Many people think they can eat whatever they want when they take these pills, but that's just not the case.

And remember that nothing takes off weight and keeps off weight like a sensible, balanced diet and exercise. Plus, no pill will help you make the emotional and lifestyle changes that you will have to make in order to lose those extra pounds.

CHAPTER 5- GETTING STARTED

Before getting started on any diet plan, it is important to have a sound plan in place.

You can lose weight in many ways. Sure you could go the supermodel route and starve yourself, but who wants to do that. There are a few things about dieting and weight loss that most experts agree upon in general. First, you need to drink a lot of water. Most individuals don't drink nearly enough water. Colas and coffee don't count! Yes, you really should drink eight 8-ounce glasses of water a day - maybe more, depending on your weight. Water is a natural appetite suppressant. If you drink a full glass of water before beginning your meal, your stomach simply doesn't hold as much food.

No, you will not gain weight from drinking a lot of water. It's when you don't drink enough water throughout the day, your body gets dehydrated. When it does finally get water, it holds onto it and stores it for a future need. That's when we feel swollen, and bloated with water weight. However, if you give your body enough water on a regular basis, it releases it naturally. Drinking enough water gives you the benefit of hydration and fullness. You should always eat a balanced meal. This might be the one thing we learned in elementary school that we really can use in our adult life – the basic food groups. Proteins and carbohydrates are essential to a healthy meal. Carbohydrates are the main source of energy in our diet, and proteins burn fat. At a bare minimum, each meal should consist of a protein and a carbohydrate. DO NOT skip meals. One of the worst things we can do, in our attempt to lose weight, is to skip a meal. I've seen it countless times: Motivated to lose weight, an individual decides to eat just twice a day. But your metabolism needs the consistency of regular meals. With erratic eating schedules, the body thinks it's starving. So, everything it takes in – it stores as fat to be used for energy. Finally, exercise. You just can't lose weight when you maintain a sedentary lifestyle. People who exercise live longer and feel better. And, they lose weight quicker. But, keep it simple.

Thomas Jefferson said, "The sovereign invigorator of the body is exercise, and of all the exercises walking is the best."

It's never too late to get in shape. We'll give you a whole separate section on exercise, but you don't have to join a gym and become the next famous body builder. There's plenty of ways you can get enough exercise to aid in your weight loss efforts.

Of course, there is a simple formula to help calculate weight loss: consume fewer calories than what you burn every day. For example, if you consume 2000 calories per day and you burn 2500 calories per day, you will lose weight.

You might just say "Why don't I just cut down on my calories intake considerably, hence I don't really have to burn many calories to lose weight?" Well that would be starving yourself and is not a good idea at all. This will make you weaker, hungrier and you will eat quite a lot after. Your body needs food and calories to get energy. You need to eat enough so as not to starve yourself and be able to burn these calories and more after. On the other hand, if you burn out the exact same amount of calories that you take, you will stay the same.

The secret to losing weight without going hungry is to make the right food choices. You need to choose foods that are low in calories but can satisfy your stomach so you don't become hungry.

We found a very interesting study that illustrates how the way we eat affects our weight. It was performed by New Zealand's

University of Auckland in 1999. The researchers divided male participants into three groups. Each group was put on a diet with different fat percentages (their total daily calories were composed of 60, 40 or 20-percent fat) but no calorie limits. The men were told to eat as much they wanted from the food choices they were allowed.

As expected, the men eating the 20-percent fat diets lost weight because they were consuming fewer calories. Fat contains nine calories per gram compared to four calories per gram for carbohydrates or protein. Therefore, the more fat a food contains the more calories it will have. However, in spite of the lower calorie diet, the men in this group were not at all hungry.

What the researchers discovered was that the men in the low-fat group unconsciously compensated by choosing foods that weighed the same as the men in the higher-fat groups and, therefore, were not hungry. What this suggests is that the weight of the food you eat may play a more important role than fat or calories in satisfying your hunger. In other words, you may not need to eat high-calorie or high-fat foods to feel full but your stomach has to feel the weight of a certain amount of food. There are several other studies suggesting that people tend to eat the same weight of food daily, regardless of the fat or calories that the meals contain. It's almost as if your stomach has an internal scale with a pre-determined weight that has to be reached for you to be satisfied and not hungry.

This may explain the rationale behind drinking a glass of water or having a bowl of soup before eating to cut down on your appetite. It may also explain why people can go on a low fat diet and yet gain weight if the majority of their food choices come from starchy food that is highly processed and low in fiber.

You can eat many slices of fluffy white bread before you feel full while eating two slices of whole wheat multigrain bread already makes you feel like you swallowed the whole loaf. Eating high fiber foods like oatmeal helps you eat fewer calories (seven ounces of oatmeal only has 120 calories) without going hungry.

So how do you choose the right foods?

CHAPTER 6- WHAT TO EAT

All foods have to be had in moderation. To lose weight effectively cut back on eating lots of sweets, but do not eliminate it completely as that can lead to binging.

If you are trying to lose weight, choose food based on their weight-to-calorie ratio. You want to eat food that weighs a lot but has few calories and avoid food that is light in weight but hefty in calories.

Fruits and vegetables are the big winners in the heavy weight-low calorie department, according to Tufts University. They weigh a lot because of their fiber and water content and yet do not have many calories. For example, one cup of cantaloupe or 'melon' weighs 5.5 ounces but only has 56 calories. A cup of cooked spinach weighs six ounces but only has 42 calories.

Now, compare that to six cups of buttered popcorn that only weighs three ounces and contains 420 calories or, even worse, one ounce of potato chips that has 152 calories (if you ate four ounces, you would be inviting 608 calories to feel at home in your fat cells). That's what I call "small but terrible".

Most snack food doesn't weigh much but sure have a lot of calories. This means you can eat a lot of them without feeling full and without realizing it take in many excess calories that you don't need.

Most cookies weigh ½ ounce and contain 50 calories. Eat six cookies and you only have three ounces of weight but you've racked up 300 calories. 1.5 ounces of a chocolate bar contain 220 calories. A small croissant only weighs two ounces but has 230 calories.

Angela Turner

According to the New Zealand University study, food that is light in weight but high in calories is probably the worst kind of food to eat if you are trying to lose weight. It's sort of like 'double jeopardy' - you are still hungry but you have already eaten many calories.

Choose lower-fat choices of the same weight food. There can be a world of difference between the caloric consumption of two people eating the same weight and type of food. How is this possible? Easy, if you consider the way the food is cooked or prepared.

Here are some examples (all of them weigh 3.5 ounces). Boiled potatoes have 62 calories compared to french fried potatoes with 328 calories. Sardines in tomato sauce contain 127 calories while sardines in oil have 372. Tuna flakes in water have 95 calories while tuna flakes in oil have 309. You get the picture.

Avoid the "light weight-high calorie" way of dieting. I know many people who don't want to eat regular sized meals because they think that if their stomach feels heavy, they are eating a lot of calories. Therefore, they think that by eating something light like crackers, they will lose weight. What they don't realize is that just because a food is light doesn't automatically mean it contains few calories. One could easily eat nine crackers (420 calories) and still not feel full because nine crackers only weigh three ounces. Believe it or not but you could have a satisfying meal of ½ cup steamed rice, a cup of cooked spinach, a small piece of fish, and a cup of cantaloupe for less calories. This complete meal would weigh a satisfying 18.5 ounces and only "cost" you 378 calories. By making the right food choices, you can cut down on unnecessary calories without starving yourself and feeling deprived. You should also cut down somewhat on your carbs, but don't cut them out completely! Because effective weight loss depends on exercise and activity, without some carbs in your diet, you won't have the energy you'll need to effectively burn off calories.

What you do need to do is begin with a "baseline diet" that dictates at least half of your calories come from vegetables, fruits, natural starches, and whole grains. The rest of your diet should consist of low-fat proteins like fish, chicken, and lean beef.

You need to balance out your carbs with your protein stay away from those carbs at night. Periodically, you want to take "carb-up" days to get your energy levels up. When we talk about protein, many people wonder just how much is enough or how much is too much. In general, experts say you should eat 1 gram of protein for every pound of body weight per meal.

That might seem like a ridiculously large amount of protein, but remember, we're talking about LEAN proteins. Plus, eating protein speeds up your metabolism and accelerates weight loss.

This might be a good time to talk about portion sizes. As a general rule of thumb, you should never eat a serving that is larger than your clenched fist. The good news about this is that you'll be able to eat enough to get full without overdoing it.

Cravings might be the worst part about weight loss. Let's say you love chocolate chip cookies like I do. If you're craving a chocolate chip cookie, denying that craving will only make it stronger.

Instead of not having the cookie, go ahead, just don't overdo it. Simply have one instead of three. You can indulge in your favorite foods as long as you keep it within reason.

Most experts agree that the traditional three square meals a day shouldn't be part of a healthy diet. In fact, you should eat more meals every day. Doesn't that sound like great news?!

The idea here is that you overeat when you are overly hungry. To combat that hunger, you should eat more meals with smaller portions rather than fewer meals with larger portions.

For women, it is recommended you eat five meals a day and for men, you should eat six. Try to make these meals a minimum of 2 hours apart to insure you don't get too hungry.

The benefits will reveal themselves. By doing this, you are accomplishing the following benefits:

- Faster metabolic rate

- Higher energy

- Less storage of body fat due to the smaller portions

- Reduced hunger and cravings

- Steadier blood sugar and insulin levels

- More calories available for muscle growth

- Better absorption and utilization of the nutrients in your food But you need to make sure you eat the right kinds of foods.

CHAPTER 7- FORBIDDEN FOODS FOR WEIGHT LOSS

Certain foods do have to be avoided during the weight loss process.

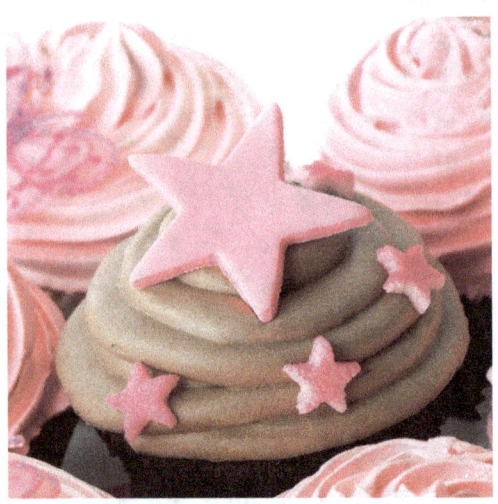

We can't possibly cover all of the foods that are acceptable to eat when you are trying to lose weight. Common sense can tell you that French fries are a no-no and an apple is great.

What we've decided to do is concentrate on those foods that you SHOULDN'T eat. Of course, this could be a long list as well, so we're going to touch on the worst and give you some possible substitutions.

Beverages

Stay away from anything with caffeine in it - don't forget that many sodas have caffeine. Caffeine has the same insulin-stimulating, weight-loss-inhibiting effect as aspartame. Unfortunately, this includes coffee. Stick to decaffeinated sodas, teas, and coffees.

Along the same lines, cut out any beverage that contains aspartame (Nutra Sweet), high fructose corn syrup, or refined sugar. Since you need to drink a lot of water in order to lose weight, try water with a slice of lemon or lime in it. It can be very refreshing and very satisfying! Alcohol is a no-no in any weight loss plan. It's OK to have a glass of wine with dinner, just don't drink the whole bottle. There's no better way to pack on the pounds than to drink excessive amounts of alcohol – even the ones that claim they have fewer calories. Moderation is the key with alcoholic beverages!

Boxed Pre-Packaged Foods

In general, you should stay away from a lot of these products. If the ingredients are not pronounceable, you should avoid them. In other words, anything with a lot of chemicals on the ingredient list are not going to be good for your diet.

White rice, while very filling, contains starches that can inhibit your weight loss. Stick to brown rice instead. Pasta mixes are usually also not good because of the starches they contain. Stick to whole grain pastas instead. They taste just as good and are much better for you!

Breads

For the same reasons as pasta and white rice, white breads should also be avoided. Whole grain breads provide you with the carbohydrates you need and are less processed than the white breads. Be sure the bread you choose is made with whole wheat flour instead of just wheat flour. Believe me, it makes a difference.

If you love Mexican food, stick to whole wheat flour tortillas or corn tortillas when you choose your burritos, enchiladas, or soft tacos.

Canned and Jar Foods

Again, anything that is canned or jarred needs to be free of excessive chemicals. If the label contains ingredients with more than four syllables or are hyphenated, it won't be good for your diet.

Chicken broth can be very fatty, so stay away. So are many soup mixes. The good news is that there are plenty of light or low fat choices out there. These are the ones you should choose.

Commercially-made tomato sauces or tomato based sauces contain ridiculously huge amounts of sugar and salt. A better choice is to make these sauces yourself where you can control what goes into it. We'll have a recipe later in the book for you to do just that!

Do not eat canned fruit or canned vegetables. If it's been canned, it's been cooked thus it loses some of its most beneficial nutrients. They can also contain processed or refined sugars, so stick to fresh fruits and veggies instead. If you have to have a little oil to cook your foods in, choose extra virgin olive oil over the vegetable or corn based oils.

Meats

Choose only lean meats to get your protein intake. It's commonly known that you should try to stay away from red meats like beef. Of course, if you're like me and love your steak, choose a lean cut and don't make the portion any larger than your clenched fist.

Choose fresh fish instead of canned and be sure it's of the lower fat variety. This includes salmon, tilapia, and cod. Don't bread your fish either, broil it or grill it to get rid of any residual fat that might remain.

White meat chicken breasts are better than dark meat because the darker meat contains more fat. The same applies to turkey.

Tuna is always a good choice – even if it's canned. Just be sure to get the tuna canned in water – not oil!

Dairy

Skim milk should be your first choice over whole milk or two percent. Avoid drinking too much milk, however, because it naturally contains some fats that can turn into unnecessary fat on you!

Unfortunately, cheese on a diet is also a big no-no. However, you can find low-fat or fat-free cheese in most grocery stores, so always pick these first. But use it sparingly!

Eggs are all right on your diet, but you're better off to use only the whites instead of including the yolks. Egg substitutes are a great way to get your egg fix, so look for these in the store as well.

Fat-free sour cream is alright in moderation, but try to substitute with plain yogurt instead.

Vegetables and Fruits

Almost all fresh vegetables are good for you. It's a generally accepted belief that you can eat all the vegetables you want and still lose weight. That's pretty much true – as long as they're prepared the correct way. It's always best to steam veggies. You can also drizzle them with a little olive oil and bake them in the oven or – even better – roast them on the grill! Yummy!

Be careful of eating too many fruits that contain a lot of natural sugars like oranges and peaches. Because the sugar is naturally there, it's not horribly bad for you, but you don't want to overload on sugars because it can be converted to fat.

One big thing you must do when you decide that you want to lose weight is to immediately clean the cupboards and refrigerator getting rid of all the foods that can inhibit your diet. That means get rid of the chips, processed sugar, canned fruits, etc.

Don't throw them away – give them to a local food bank. Believe me; they'll be happy to get whatever you have to offer – diet friendly or not!

Once you do that, you get to go shopping! Don't dread it! Just shop smart!

CHAPTER 8- GROCERY SHOPPING FOR YOUR DIET

When shopping for foods it is best to avoid the aisles with pre-packaged and pre-processed foods. Stick to the aisles with fresh organic produce.

The first rule of shopping when you're trying to lose weight is to shop with a list. This is extremely important, because you don't want to fall prey to the natural instincts of wanting to grab those cookies that are there on that special display at the end of aisle four. Stick to that list faithfully, too.

Plan before you shop. Of course! If you didn't plan, how could you have the list, right? You need to decide what your meals are going to be and what ingredients you will need to prepare them. Be sure to include portion sizes when planning your meals.

Don't just plan for dinners. Remember, you will be eating several smaller meals per day, so include all the meals in your agenda.

When you first start shopping for your weight loss trip, it might be a good idea to take along someone to keep you in check as you stroll the aisles. This needs to be someone who knows your struggles with weight loss and who can support this journey with you.

They need to be your shopping police, so don't blame them if they take those cookies back out of your cart. Remember, you want their support, so don't blame them. Give them permission to keep you focused. You may also want to involve them in the planning process as well so they have a better idea of what exactly you are trying to accomplish.

We can't stress this next point enough: EAT BEFORE YOU GO SHOPPING! It's a well-known fact that if you are hungry when you go to the grocery store, you will be more prone to making impulse purchases that aren't good for you because it sounds so yummy!

Learn how to read labels. As we've said before, you have to avoid products that have ingredients that will be bad for your diet. Look at the fat content, the sugar content, the salt content, etc. Be sure that you are buying weight friendly foods that you will be able to eat and not have to worry about when they're in your cupboard. Avoid convenience foods. Even though they are easy to fix and taste pretty good, these types of foods often contain additional calories, fats, and carbohydrates that you just don't need. If you find yourself drawn to the diet dinners in the frozen food section, be sure to read the ingredients before you buy!

You will always be better off if you prepare your meals yourself. That means plan to cook from scratch. If you think you don't have the time, think again. We'll give you some great recipes that you can either make ahead of time or that you can prepare in less than 30 minutes! When you cook your own meals, you will have complete control over what you put into your food (salt, sugar, etc.) plus they will taste a lot better than convenience foods.

While it may seem painfully obvious, we can't stress enough – don't buy foods with empty calories. Those foods include chips, cookies, candy, etc. You don't need the temptation, and they provide absolutely NO nutritional value for you at all, so avoid them like the plague! No matter how good you eat, you will have to exercise in order to lose weight.

CHAPTER 9- EXERCISE AND WEIGHT LOSS

Apart from dieting, exercise can help speed up the weight loss process. It also helps to tone the body as the pounds are shed.

Even with those "miracle" diet pills, you still cannot lose weight without increasing your physical activity. Exercising in some form will help to burn calories that can be converted into fat and extra weight. This is why you need to devise an effective workout plan that will fit into your abilities and interests.

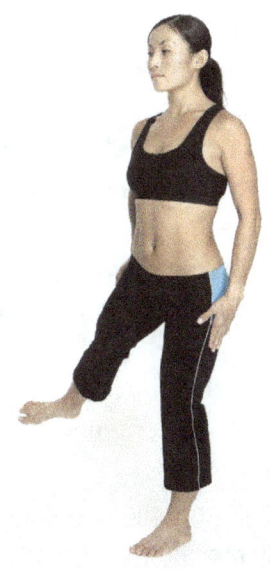

Most people don't really like to exercise. For them, it seems too much like work. And it is work, but it doesn't have to be tedious work. There are ways to exercise doing things that you love to do.

First, you need to choose an activity that you enjoy.

Do you like riding your bike as the sun sets in the sky? Maybe swimming is more your idea of fun. Even a good round of golf can be a great form of exercise – but only if you leave the cart in the cart barn!

Once you find that activity, you need to pursue it at a minimum of three times a week for at least 30 minutes at a time. The more you exercise, the more calories you will burn, but you don't have to be fanatical about it! Start slowly then increase your level when you feel stronger until you are at a point where you think you are at a high level of intensity. It's OK to rest at intervals to recharge your batteries, but get back up to that level again until your workout is complete.

The ideal exercise plan is going to involve some form of aerobic exercise sustained for 30 minutes at a time. This could be in the form of an aerobics class or something as simple as taking a walk. This will get your heart pumping effectively so that your body can burn the calories that you have consumed!

When should you do this type of workout? Believe it or not, there is a best time to perform your cardio workout for best results.

We want to tell you that the important part about exercise is that you get out and do it! No matter when you exercise, you will burn fat and calories as long as it's a good workout. But to get the maximum benefit, try exercising in the morning before you eat your first meal. Early morning aerobic exercising on an empty stomach has three benefits over working out later in the day. First, your levels of stored carbohydrates and muscle are at a low when you first get up in the morning. This is because during the night, your body is burning any calories that were consumed at dinner the previous evening by performing bodily functions that occur even while we sleep. As a result, you'll wake up with lower carb levels and lower blood sugar levels which is the optimum environment for burning fat instead of carbs.

How does this work? It's actually quite simple. Carbohydrates are your body's primary and preferred energy source. When this source is in short supply, your body must tap into its secondary energy resource: body fat. If you do your exercise workout after eating, the body will burn off the carbohydrates you've consumed first. It'll take a little longer to get to that fat you need to burn. A second benefit to doing exercise in the morning is called the "afterburn" effect. You'll not only be burning fat during your workout, but that fat burn will continue on even after your workout is finished. How?

An intense session of cardio can keep your metabolism elevated for hours afterwards. Exercising at night won't give you that extra metabolic lift because once you go to sleep, your metabolism drops dramatically once you become sedentary. When you sleep, your metabolic rate is slower than at any other time of the day.

The third reason for doing early morning exercise is more emotional than anything else. Your body's endorphins are elevated when you exercise. It lifts your mood and gives you a sense of accomplishment that will likely stay with you all during the day.

That being said, exercise is something that many consider a tedious chore. We tend to procrastinate and put off doing something we consider to be less than enjoyable. If you commit yourself to morning workouts, you'll have "gotten it out of the way" freeing your mind from having to do it later. This can create guilt and stress and affect your whole day – don't let it! Plus, you are more likely to blow off exercising later in the day because you are tired or just don't feel like it.

You might find it difficult to get up and exercise first thing in the morning. Not everyone is a "morning person". So how do you motivate yourself to get up and get moving? First, remember that you are trying to lose weight. You have a goal that you are trying to achieve. That should remain in the forefront of your mind. If you stay focused on your goal, the motivation should come. Think back to a time when you tackled a difficult task and finished it. Remember how great you felt afterwards. Completing any challenge can give you a "buzz". When that task is physically demanding, that "buzz" is both psychological and physiological. That's because your body releases endorphins into your system. Endorphins are opiate-like hormones that are hundreds of times more powerful than the strongest morphine. Except for endorphins are made by YOU, not a laboratory. Endorphins create a natural high that can make you positively euphoric! Endorphins can reduce stress, improve your mood, increase your circulation, and relieve pain. This "high" you feel is partly psychological too. When you get up early and get your workout done, you'll feel a sense of completion that will kick start your day and get it off on the right foot! You will have a sense of completion and accomplishment that will stay with you throughout your day. You'll feel happy and less stressed when you know that this difficult task is already behind you and you can enjoy what the day has to offer you!

So, you know that exercise is essential to any weight loss program, but what kind of exercise should you do? What kind of exercise is best? We've already said that you should choose something you love to do so that exercising doesn't seem so tedious, but maybe you're wondering whether or not you should get into the gym and lift the big weights or simply take a walk to get your aerobic exercise in.

There really is no cut and dried answer to this question. Whether you want to bust out the old Tae-Bo tapes, plunk down a bunch of money on a treadmill, or just put on some music and do some leg lifts on your living room floor, the important thing is that you do exercise. Let's look at the calorie burning that occurs in certain types of exercises.

The numbers below reflect the number of calories you burn for 20 minutes of participation in different exercises. We should all aim to take 30 minutes of moderate exercise 5 days a week. This can be a mixture of all types of physical activity, anything that makes you slightly out of breath and raises your heart rate slightly.

This table doesn't only show values for organized exercises, but also for more enjoyable pass times, like walking, dancing and gardening - which many of us enjoy to do.

CHAPTER 10- ACTIVITY CALORIES

Certain activities help to burn more calories than other activities. One simply has to look up the information and determine which options work best for you.

Leisurely walk 80

Dancing 120

Cycling 160

Running 325

Aerobics 140

Weights 140

Cleaning 125

Driving 35

Swimming 100

Tennis 120

Rowing 378

Golf 118

Circuit Training 260

Skipping 100

Gardening 160

Skiing 130

Mowing The Lawn 125

Fishing 114

Basketball 258

Bowling 108

Riding a Horse 255

Walking Downstairs 210

Walking Upstairs 300-500

Roller Skating 315

Having Sex 350

Almost any activity can be a fat burning activity – as you can see from the above chart. Yes, even having sex can burn calories! However, keep in mind that the number given above is for 30 minutes of activity! Generally, men tend to burn more calories during sex than women do, but if you're going to incorporate some love making into your workout regimen (and we hope you do!), be an active participant – don't just lay there and think you're burning calories.

CHAPTER 11- EXERCISE ROUTINES

There are some simple yet effective exercises that can help to speed up the metabolism and burn those calories.

So here are a few suggestions for some exercises you can do at home. The best part about exercising at home is that you can do these exercises even while you watch television. No need to give up your favorite programs to get active, just get on the floor and try this workout:

- Jumping Jacks - 1 minute
- Squats – 15 to 20 times
- Push-Ups – As many as you can
- Jog in place making your foot hit your butt – 1 minute
- Superman – lay flat on the floor on stomach with hands stretched out to the side. Lift legs and chest off the floor and hold for 30 second – 15 to 20 times
- High Knees – jog in place lifting your knees as high as you can – 1 minute
- Lunges – feet flat on the floor, step forward with alternating feet – 15 to 20 times
- Torso Rotation/Twists – 20 times each direction
- Side Bends/Reaches – 20 times each direction
- Wall Sit – Squat against a wall with your back flat on the wall – sit as long as you can hold it and that's it! Do this every day and feel the benefits.

CHAPTER 12- TONING EXERCISES

A toned body is a healthy one. There is no need to do extreme weight lifting to achieve this and it will also help sculpt the body as the pounds are being shed.

Need some more exercises? No problem! Here are three exercises that can be used to tighten thighs, buttocks, and stomach areas.

Outer Thigh Lift – Lying on your right side with your hips and ankles in line with your shoulders, slowly lift your leg as high as possible, hold, then return to starting position. Do 10 repetitions and then switch sides.

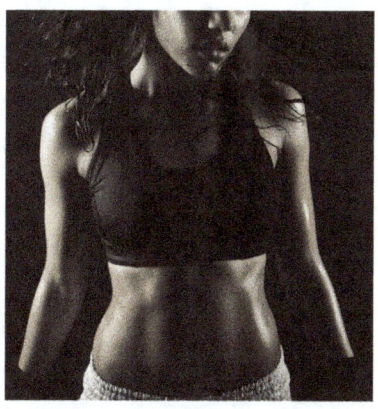

Inner Thigh Lift – Lie on your left side with your hips and ankles in line with your shoulders, and your right knee bent at a 90 degree angle. Slowly lift your left leg as high as possible, hold, then return to starting position. Do 10 repetitions and then switch sides

Abdominal Crunches – Lying on your back with your knees bent and your hands behind your head, slowly curl your shoulders up putting your chin to your chest. Pause then slowly return to starting position. Do 10 repetitions of these.

Of course, these are toning exercises that will help target problem areas. One problem area many women have is cellulite in the thigh area and other places. Here are some exercises to perform that will help those cellulite areas.

CHAPTER 13- EXERCISES FOR CELLULITE

Many females are concerned with the amount of cellulite that they have on their bodies and will do almost anything to get rid of it.

Lying on your side, do 10 repetitions of each of the following exercises:

- Bring both knees forward so your hips are at a 90 degree angle. Straighten your top leg out in front of you while maintaining the 90 degree hip placement. Lift the top leg slowly up about three feet off the ground and then lower.
- Straighten both legs so your body is in a straight line.
- Tilt your hips forward slightly. Lift your top leg about three feet off the ground then lower.
- Put your top leg out in front of you on the ground.
- Move your bottom leg forward slightly. Lift the bottom leg 8-12 inches off the ground and down.
- Repeat all three exercises on the other side.

On your elbows and knees, do 10 repetitions of each of the following exercises:

- Extend one leg straight back with your toe on the ground. Lift that leg up to the ceiling and then back down. Switch legs.
- Lift your knee off the floor. Extend that same heel back and up so that your leg is pointing toward the ceiling and then bring the knee back into you. Switch legs.

From a standing position, do 10 repetitions of the following exercises:

- Start with your feet together. Step out in front of you in a lunge position. Touch the ground with the opposite hand. Come back up and step to the starting position. Switch legs.
- Put one foot on a step or prop that is 12-18 inches high. Slowly step up and down with the other foot. Switch legs.

You can increase the intensity of this workout by going through it more than once or increasing the amount of repetitions.

CHAPTER 14- WALKING FOR WEIGHT LOSS

Walking can help person to shed weight as well. this can be done to build up the stamina as well until running can be done.

Exercises are good for your workout program because they help tone flabby muscles while also burning calories. But aerobic exercise is best to burn fat. A great way to get an aerobic workout is to walk.

Walking is the easiest and most effective exercise we can use in our workout routine. But you need to know more than one foot in front of the other to get the most from walking as aerobic exercise.

Because of how the body draws on fat stores versus other stored energy sources, the first thing you need to do is increase the time you spend walking. While we've said that 30 minutes of exercise is good for fat burning, when you walk, you really need to bump this up to at least 45 minutes, but ideally an hour.

Obviously, it might not be possible for you to fit an hour of walking into your busy schedule, but try walking every day allowing a few days for an hour and a few days at 30 minutes. Alternate them, however. If you walk an hour on Monday, walk half an hour on Tuesday, etc. If you're only going to be walking for 30 minutes, increase your speed. A leisurely stroll isn't going to give you that aerobic workout that your body needs, so step it up a bit. But don't overdo it. If you can't talk and walk, you're over-exerting yourself and you should back off a bit. You can also introduce some type of weight for you to carry when you walk. This could be something simple like a small weight, or you can go to the pantry and pull out a couple of cans of corn! Keep them in your hands as you walk and move your arms back and forth in your strides. Adding weight will also help tone your arms – an added perk!

If you're walking outdoors, perhaps in your neighborhood, take along a walk-man and play some upbeat music to keep you walking. Not only is it entertaining, it keeps you going as well!

And remember, that all walking counts – even if it's during a shopping trip to the mall!

CHAPTER 15- OTHER FORMS OF EXERCISE

There really is no excuse for not doing some form of exercise as the options are numerous. All you have to do is find some that you would enjoy doing and get started!

There are all kinds of ways you can work exercise into your life. You can workout anywhere doing all sort of things. Playing with children, for example is a great way to get some exercise. When you get down on the floor and play "horsey", you are giving yourself a heck of a workout – and it is fun for the kids!

Throw a ball around in the backyard and really get into it! Jump on a trampoline, or just play tag! Exercise like this not only give you the physical benefits, it can remind you of the joy of youth and put a real smile on your face! At work, take the stairs instead of the elevator. When you park in a parking lot, park as far away from the door as possible so you have to walk further. Use your imagination and you will find ways to exercise almost anywhere!

Many people love the idea of being in a gym surrounded by sweaty people who are lifting weights and using the stair-stepping machine. If this is what you like, by all means, get into the gym.

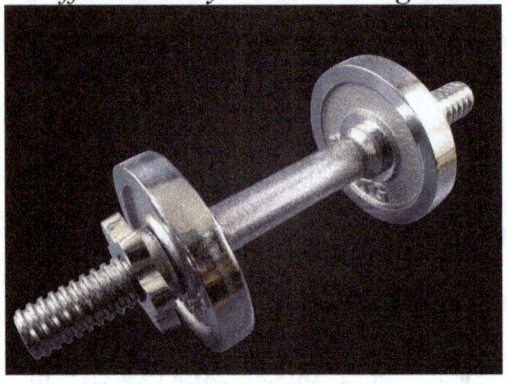

Weight training gives you the opportunity to sculpt your body by pushing your muscles toward working harder than they normally would.

We suggest that you get the advice of someone in the gym like the trainer or owner to give you some exercises to start out with. They will be the experts in the field for you and will know what works when you're just beginning a weight training program. They can also help guide you when it's time for you to "step up" your regimen. Aerobics classes are another great way to get a terrific workout. You can find classes like these in many, many places, but mostly in gyms and workout studios. Keep in mind that there will be a fee to take these classes, but it might very well be worth it to have the camaraderie that comes with other people sweating along with you! We highly recommend looking into taking water aerobics. Exercising in the water has so many benefits. You have less stress and strain on your joints, plus the natural resistance of the water will work your muscles more than if you were taking a class "on land".

Water aerobics can be done by just about anyone –young and old alike. It's a great alternative to strength training and you won't have the problem of excessive sweating that many of us just hate! You'll get an amazing workout and it'll be fun too!

Many people – the Hollywood elite included – are beginning to advocate Pilates as a very effective weight loss method. This exercise regimen was developed in the early 20th century, but has just now come to global popularity. Pilates is more than exercise program, it is based on the principles of many different types of movements. It takes some of its movements from yoga, acrobats, stretching, and more. Plus, Pilates concentrates a lot on the mind as an exercise tool.

We can't tell you how to do Pilates because it's so involved. That would be a whole other book to write! But there are many helpful tools out there that can help you with a Pilates program if you think that the route you want to go. Look for online web sites, videos, and classes in your area. Once you learn the basic movements, you can then practice them on your own!

So now we know about exercising in order to lose weight, but let's get back to the most important hurdle in trying to lose weight – the food!

CHAPTER 16- COUNTING CALORIES

Though counting calories is recommended to keep track of weight loss, it can become an obsessive task so one has to be careful.

Many people think that when they decide it's time to lose weight, they have to count every single calorie that touches their lips. This really isn't necessary. In fact, it could become quite tedious and cause you to give up. So how do you know how many calories you've taken in during a 24 hour period? Estimate! Count portions instead of each individual calorie. This is where effective meal planning comes in!

When you know approximately how many calories are in that piece of bread and 2 ounces of tuna, you can have a general idea of how many calories you're consuming when you eat a tuna sandwich.

If you insist on tracking all of your calories, you'll have to be diligent about reading labels and eating only the portions that the label gives calories for. You'll also have to carry around a small notebook to jot down what you've eaten so you can assign a calorie value for reference. A much easier way might be to utilize a spreadsheet that lists your planned meals along with their caloric content. Be sure to include other particulars such as protein content, carbs, and fat grams as well. Then print it out and post it on your refrigerator to give yourself something to aspire to.

Almost all packaged foods will contain information about the caloric content of those foods, but what about those fruits and vegetables you consume. Maybe we should give you some ideas!

Food Portion Calories

Apples 1 medium 125

Asparagus 4 spears 15

Avocado 1 305

Banana 1 105

Beef Roast, Lean 3 oz. 205

Beef Sirloin Steak 3 oz. 240

Blackberries 1 cup 75

Broccoli 1 cup 45

Cabbage 1 cup 30

Cantaloupe ½ melon 95

Carrots 1 30

Celery 1 stalk 5

Cherries 10 50

Chicken, Roasted

Breast

3 oz. 140

Chicken, Fried

Breast

4.6 oz. 369

Yellow Corn 1 ear 85

Crab Meat 1 cup 135

Cucumber 6 slices 5

Egg, Fried 1 egg 90

Egg, Hard Boiled 1 egg 75

Egg, Scrambled 1 egg 100

Flounder, Baked 3 oz. 120

Pink Grapefruit ½ fruit 40

Ground Beef,

Broiled

3 oz. 230

Halibut, Broiled 3 oz. 140

Lamb Chop,

Broiled

2.8 oz. 235

Lamb Leg, Roasted 3 oz. 205

Lettuce 1 cup 5

Mushrooms 1 cup 20

Nectarine 1 65

Okra, Cooked 8 pods 25

Orange 1 60

Peaches 1 35

Pear 1 100

Peanuts, Salted 1 cup 71

Pepper, Green/Red 1 15

Pineapple 1 cup 75

Pistachios 1 oz. 165

Pork Chop, Broiled 2.5 oz. 165

Pork Chop, Fried 3.1 oz. 335

Pork – Ham –

Roasted

3 oz. 250

Pork Rib – Roasted 3 oz. 270

Pork Bacon 3 slices 110

Pork Sausage Link 1 link 50

Potato – Baked 1 220

Raisins 1 cup 435

Salmon – Smoked 3 oz. 150

Spinach 1 cup 10

Strawberries 1 cup 45

Sweet Potato –

Baked

1 115

Tangerine 1 35

Tomato 1 25

Turkey – Roasted 1 cup 240

Walnuts 1 cup 770

Watermelon 1 cup 50

Obviously, this is just a partial list, but it's a start for you to reference when choosing foods. As you can see, fruits and vegetables are almost all relatively low-calorie and can help you feel full without consuming a lot of calories. You will want to consume fewer calories than what you burn off in order to effectively lose weight. Keep that in mind when planning your meals.

And we can't stress this enough — read labels and take note of portion sizes! That way you can get a better idea of what you're eating.

We promised you some great low-cal recipes, so let's get to it!.

CHAPTER 17- YUMMY RECIPES

If you know what is best to eat then a smooth transition can be made to the new lifestyle where meal choices are healthier.

As the topic of this book says – you CAN lose weight without starving yourself. We've given you all kinds of tips and tricks toward achieving this on your own. Now we're going to offer up some great recipes for you to create on your own that will be diet-friendly and delicious too!

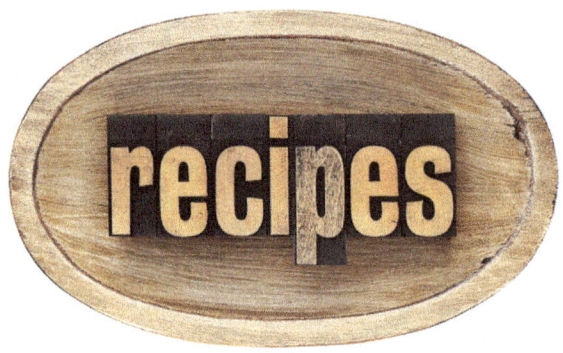

BREAKFAST

When you eat breakfast, you can always let yourself pig out on all the fresh fruit you desire, but sometimes you find yourself craving something more substantial. You CAN eat a hearty breakfast while trying to lose weight. Consider some of these great recipes!

Egg-White Omelet with Vegetable-Cheddar Filling

3 large egg whites
1 teaspoon water

Angela Turner

2 teaspoons chopped fresh dill (optional)

1/8 teaspoon salt

1/8 teaspoon freshly ground pepper

½ cup loosely packed thinly sliced fresh spinach 1 plum tomato, chopped 2 tablespoons shredded nonfat cheddar cheese Vegetable cooking spray 1. Whisk egg whites, water, dill (if using), salt, and pepper together in a medium bowl until soft peaks form. Toss spinach, tomato, and cheddar together in a small bowl. 2. Lightly coat an omelet pan or small skillet with cooking spray and heat over medium heat 1 minute. Pour egg mixture into pan and cook until eggs begin to set on bottom. 3. Spread filling over half of omelet, leaving a ½-inch border and reserving 1 tablespoon mixture for garnish. Lift up omelet at edge nearest handle and fold in half, slightly off-center, so filling peeks out. Cook 2 minutes. Slide omelet onto a serving plate and garnish with reserved filling.

Serves: 1

Zesty Cheddar-Asparagus Quiche

1 tablespoon plain dry breadcrumbs

8 ounces small all-purpose potatoes, peeled and very thinly sliced

2 teaspoons olive oil

1 pound asparagus, trimmed

½ teaspoon salt, divided

¾ cup shredded reduced-fat sharp cheddar cheese

3 scallions, sliced

1 can (12 ounces) evaporated fat-free milk

2 large eggs

2 large egg whites

2 teaspoons butter, melted

1 teaspoon dry mustard

¼ teaspoon freshly ground pepper

Heat oven to 400°F. Coat a 9-inch pie plate with vegetable cooking spray and sprinkle with breadcrumbs. Beginning in center, arrange potato slices in slightly overlapping circles up to rim. Lightly brush with olive oil and press down gently. Bake 10 minutes. 2. Set 8 to 12 asparagus spears aside. Cut remaining spears into 1-inch pieces.

Sprinkle crust with ¼ teaspoon salt and ¼ cup cheddar. Cover with asparagus pieces, then sprinkle with scallions and another ¼ cup cheese. Arrange whole asparagus spears on top.

Beat evaporated milk, eggs, egg whites, butter, mustard, pepper, and remaining ¼ teaspoon salt in a medium bowl. Pour into pie plate and sprinkle with remaining cheddar. Bake until a knife inserted in center comes out clean, about 35 minutes.

Divide into 6 slices. One serving equals 1 slice.

Quick French Toast

1 large egg
½ teaspoon vanilla extract
¼ teaspoon cinnamon
1 packet artificial sweetener
1 tablespoon skim milk
1 slice bread

Place all ingredients except bread in a blender; blend until combined.

Pour egg mixture into a shallow bowl. Place bread in egg mixture and soak, turning once.

Coat a nonstick skillet with vegetable cooking spray and heat over medium heat. Place bread in skillet and pour any remaining egg mixture over bread. Cook until browned on bottom; then turn over to brown other side.

Golden Pancakes

1 c uncooked whole-grain oats
6 egg whites
1 c fat-free cottage cheese
¼ tsp vanilla extract
¼ tsp ground cinnamon
2 packets sugar substitute
½ c sugar-free maple syrup
¼ c mixed berries

Lightly coat a nonstick skillet or griddle with cooking spray and place over medium heat 2. In a blender, combine oats, egg whites, cottage cheese, vanilla, cinnamon, and sugar substitute. Blend on medium speed about 1 minute until smooth.

Pour batter about ¼ c at a time onto hot skillet. Cook pancake until bubbly on top and dry around the edges –about 3 minutes. Turn and cook the other side until golden brown – about 2 more minutes 4. While pancakes are cooking, microwave maple syrup until warm – about 20 seconds 5. Place a portion of pancakes on 2 separate plates, top with warm maple syrup and mixed berries.

Turkey Bacon Quiche

6 strips lean turkey bacon
3 eight-inch whole wheat tortillas
3 whole eggs
8 egg whites (or 1 c egg substitute)
½ c skim milk
½ c low-fat sour cream
¾ reduced-fat shredded cheddar cheese

1 c broccoli florets

Preheat oven to 350 degrees

Cook turkey bacon according to package directions.

Set aside to cool.

Lightly coat a 9-inch pie plate with cooking spray. Overlap 2 tortillas and cut the third one in half to form a crust 4. In a large mixing bowl, beat whole eggs and egg whites with a fork or whisk until well blended. Mix skim milk and sour cream into the eggs. 5. Chop cooked turkey bacon into bite size pieces 6. Add turkey, bacon, cheese, and broccoli to blended egg mixture, combine thoroughly 7. Pour egg mixture into tortilla-lined pie plate and bake for about 50 minutes. Tap the edge of the pie plate. When the filling is set and moist but not liquidy, it is done.

Cool for 10 minutes before slicing into portions. Whole wheat toast or English muffins are also good choices as are low-fat or no-fat yogurt. Just keep portion sizes to what we've talked about before.

LUNCH

Traditionally, lunch is the middle meal of the day when we eat three squares. Since you're trying to lose weight without starving yourself, experts recommend that you eat several smaller meals, so consider lunches, your daytime meals.

Obviously, you can have sandwiches – on whole wheat bread, of course! Be sure anything you put between those two pieces of bread is lean and diet-friendly. Tuna is a great and filling sandwich, but lean roast beef, no-fat cheese, and chicken salad is also a good sandwich. You can also opt for the traditional salad. Make sure you don't top it with anything that will sabotage your weight loss efforts. That means no cheese (unless it's non-fat or low-fat), bacon bits, croutons, or garbanzo beans - and no dressing unless it's light. Try some lemon juice instead. It's refreshing and delicious!

But there are other meals you can have during the day that are much more substantial meals you can have. Try some of these recipes!

Cool Taco Salad

½ lean ground beef
1 tbsp water
2 tsp. taco seasoning mix, divided
2 whole wheat pitas
2 tbsp reduced-fat cream cheese, room temp
2 tbsp fat-free sour cream
2 tbsp salsa
1 c shredded lettuce
1 diced tomato
¼ cup reduced fat shredded cheddar cheese

Preheat oven to 400 degrees

In medium skillet, brown ground beef over medium heat until done. Drain off any fat. Add water and 1 tsp taco seasoning and simmer for 3 minutes. Removed from heat and set aside to cool slightly

Cut each pita into 8 wedges and place on baking sheet.

Bake for 7 minutes or until lightly browned

While the beef is cooling, combine the remaining taco seasoning, cream cheese, sour cream, and salsa in a small bowl. Mix well. Divide and spread this mixture evenly onto 2 small plates

Spoon a portion of the beef over the sour cream mixture and top each with half the lettuce, tomato, and cheese

Place 8 baked pita wedges on each plate

2 servings

Chicken Pita Pizza

1 whole wheat pita
¼ c low fat pizza sauce
1 portion cooked chicken breast sliced
¼ red bell pepper sliced
¼ yellow bell pepper sliced
¼ small zucchini, sliced
¼ reduced-fat shredded mozzarella cheese

Preheat oven to 425 degrees

Place the pita on a baking sheet. Spoon pizza sauce

Evenly over the pita. Top with sliced chicken, peppers, zucchini and cheese

Bake for 10-12 minutes or until the cheese is melted and the pizza is heated through

Slice and eat!

Egg Salad Sandwich

Angela Turner

4 hard boiled eggs

1 tbsp fat free salad dressing (Miracle Whip)

1 tbsp mustard

½ stalk sliced celery

¼ chopping red bell pepper

1 tsp pickle relish

1 tbsp fresh parsley

1 slice whole grain bread

1 lettuce leaf

¼ sliced avocado

Chop 1 whole egg and discard the yolks from the other 3 eggs and chop the whites

In a small mixing bowl, combine all ingredients except the bread, lettuce leaf, and avocado

Toast the bread and place on a small plate. Top with lettuce, egg salad and avocado slice

1 serving

Oriental Chicken Salad

4 portions cooked chicken (about 1 lb.) in bite size pieces

1 bag coleslaw mix

4 chopped green onions

2 tbsp light sesame oil

1/3 c rice vinegar

¼ c lite soy sauce

½ tsp ground ginger

1 cup crisp chow mein noodles

In large mixing bowl, combine cooked chicken, coleslaw mix, and green onions. In small bowl, combine sesame oil, rice vinegar, soy sauce, and ginger. Drizzle over chicken mixture and toss to coat.

Divide into 4 portions and top with chow mein noodles.

4 servings

Mile High Baked Potato

1 medium russet potato
2 tsp fat-free chicken broth
¼ c low fat cottage cheese
¼ c chopped cooked chicken
¼ c cooked broccoli
¼ c salsa
1 tbsp chopped cilantro

Pierce potato several times with fork. Place in microwave and cook on high 5-8 minutes until tender. Let stand 1 minute.

Use knife to cut an "X" in the top of the cooked potato. Press ends slightly to open potato and pour chicken broth into opening

Top potato with cottage cheese, chicken, broccoli, and salsa. Place filled potato in microwave and cook on high for 30 more seconds.

Sprinkle top with fresh cilantro.

DINNER

Many people feel that dinner is the most important meal of the day. And many of them are right. Dinner is a time for families to connect, talk about their days, and bond together as a unit.

Angela Turner

Just because you're trying to lose weight doesn't mean you have to sacrifice taste at dinner time. In fact, we're willing to be that some of these recipes will be big hits with your family and they won't even know that they fit into your diet!

Spaghetti and Meatballs

1 ½ lb. lean ground turkey
2 egg whites
½ c dry breadcrumbs
¼ water
½ finely chopped onion
2 cloves minced garlic
¼ c parsley
2 tsp dried basil
1 tsp ground black pepper
3 c low-fat marinara pasta sauce
12 oz. spaghetti
¼ c reduced-fat Parmesan cheese

Preheat oven broiler

In large mixing bowl, combine turkey, egg white, breadcrumbs, water, onion, garlic, parsley, basil and black pepper. Mix thoroughly and shape into 1 ½" diameter meatballs 3. Arrange meatballs on a baking sheet and place under broiler for 10-12 minutes turning occasionally until they are browned on all sides 4. In a large saucepan, combine sauce and meatballs. Simmer on low for about 20 minutes. 5. While the sauce is simmering, prepare spaghetti according to package directions.

Plate and top with Parmesan cheese

6 servings

Homestyle Meat Loaf

1 ½ lbs. lean ground turkey

1 chopped onion

4 egg whites

1 c salsa

¾ oats, uncooked

1 pkg. dry vegetable soup mix

¼ tsp ground black pepper

½ c ketchup

6 portions red potatoes

2 lbs. green beans

¾ cup skim milk

2 tbsp Butter Buds

Preheat oven to 350 degrees

In large mixing bowl, combine turkey, onion, egg whites, salsa, oats, soup mix, and pepper. Press mixture into 9" x 5" loaf pan and spread ketchup over top. Bake in oven until no longer pink in the center –about 60 minutes. About 25 minutes after putting the meatloaf in the oven, cut potatoes into 1" chunks. Place in large saucepan and cover with water. Bring to a boil over high heat. Reduce heat to medium and simmer until tender – about 20 minutes. Cut stems off green beans and place in a large saucepan with 1" of water. Heat to boiling over high heat. Then reduce heat and simmer uncovered for 6-8 minutes until crisp-tender. Drain 5. Remove meatloaf from oven and let sit 5 minutes before slicing.

Drain potatoes and return to pan. Mash while adding skim milk a little at a time. Add butter buds and mash vigorously until light and fluffy.

Chicken Veggie Stir Fry

Angela Turner

1 tablespoon sesame oil

1 tablespoon minced garlic

1 tablespoon minced ginger

1 tablespoon minced scallions

1 pound boneless, skinless, chicken breasts, sliced into strips

1 cup broccoli spears

1 cup julienne carrots

½ pound green beans, chopped

½ cup julienne red pepper

1 cup quartered button mushrooms

3 heads baby bok choy, chopped

Low sodium teriyaki sauce

Heat the oil in a wok over high heat. Add the garlic, ginger, and scallions. Cook until aromatic, about 2 minutes.

Add the chicken. Sauté until the edges are brown, about 3 to 4 minutes.

Add the broccoli, carrots, and green beans to the wok. Cook approximately 5 to 8 minutes, until the vegetables begin to become tender. Add the red pepper, mushrooms, bok choy, and teriyaki sauce to the wok, cook approximately 5 to 8 minutes more, or until chicken is cooked through and vegetables are done to your likeness. Taste and adjust seasonings. Serve immediately.

Chicken Fried Rice with Veggies

2 cups of cooked brown rice

1 16oz bag of mixed veggies (any kind)

1 pack of chicken breast cut up

3 table spoons soy sauce

2 eggs (1 whole, 1 egg white beaten)

Cooking spray

Cook brown rice according to package and set aside.

Cook cut up chicken breast until done and set aside.

Cook beaten eggs (scrambled style) and set aside.

Cook mixed veggies according to package. 5. Spray large skillet with cooking spray, add chicken, eggs, and veggies. Stir and cook until heated through well.

Add the 3 tablespoons of soy sauce (or according to taste) to mixture in skillet. Cook for about 10 minutes to make sure it is heated through.

Beef Stroganoff

1+ pounds of top bottom roast (or sirloin)
1 8oz container of fat free sour cream
1-2 tbsp(s) of beef granules or powder
1 tbsp of flour

Whole Wheat Pasta

Veggies are optional. Recommended: Mushrooms, broccoli 1. Cut your beef into cubes or strips (if you use the round bottom roast, it is best to tenderize it). Place the beef into a pan that is sprayed with cooking spray. Cook until the beef is slightly brown (10-15 mins).

While your beef is browning, combine 8oz of sour cream, a tbsp of flour and 1-2 tbsp(s) of beef granules or powder. Mix them together (will look light brown). After beef is slightly brown, pour the sour cream mix over it. Stir and let it cook for about 8-10 mins.

While this is cooking, boil water and cook pasta. When finished place one serving of pasta on a plate and cover with meat and sauce.

Jambalaya

½ cup chopped Celery
½ cup diced Onion
½ cup diced Green Pepper
1.5 cups of diced Fat-Free Ham
1.5 cups of diced cooked boneless/skinless Chicken Breast
½ cup Chicken Broth
1 14 oz can of Diced Tomatoes (not drained) or 2 medium fresh diced tomatoes
1 tbsp Hot Sauce
1-2 tsp Cajun Seasoning
1-2 tsp Dried Jalapeño Pepper
½ cup Brown Rice (uncooked)

In a non-stick pot, or one sprayed with cooking spray, sauté Celery, Onion, and Green Pepper until Onion is tender.

Add Broth, Tomatoes, meat, and seasonings.

Bring to a boil for 5 minutes stirring frequently.

Add rice and simmer for 15 minutes stirring frequently until rice is cooked and consistency is as desired.

Chicken Noodle Soup

2 tbsp. olive oil
1 chopped onion
4 carrots peeled and chopped
4 chopped celery stalks

4 bay leaves

½ tsp ground black pepper

12 c fat-free chicken broth

2 c water

2 lb. chicken breast cut into bite-size pieces

1 lb. whole wheat or no yolk noodles

2 tbsp chopped dill

Heat olive oil in a large pot over medium heat. Add chopped onion and sauté for about 4 min.

Add carrots, celery, bay leaves, black pepper, chicken broth and water. Bring to a boil over high heat

Add chicken and bring back to coil

Add noodles and simmer until tender – about 8 minutes. Reduce heat to low

Remove bay leaves and stir in parsley and dill

8 servings

Chicken Enchiladas

1 lb. cooked and shredded chicken breast

4 sliced green onions

2 tbsp chopped cilantro

1 minced jalapeno

3 cans green enchilada sauce

8 corn tortillas

1 c reduced-fat shredded cheddar cheese

½ c salsa

½ c light sour cream

1 diced tomato

Angela Turner
¼ c sliced black olives

Preheat oven to 350 degrees. Lightly coat a 9" x 13" baking dish with cooking spray

Lightly coat a large skillet with cooking spray and place over a medium-high heat. Add green onion, cilantro, and jalapeno. Sauté for 2 min. Add chicken and 1 can of enchilada sauce. Cook, stirring occasionally until heated through – about 5 minutes

Pour the other 2 cans of enchilada sauce in a medium bowl and microwave until warm – about 2 minutes.

Dip each tortilla in the heated sauce and fill with 1/8 of the chicken mixture. Roll up and place seam-side down in the baking dish

Pour remaining heated sauce over enchiladas and sprinkle with cheese. Bake until heated through and cheese is melted – about 15 minutes.

Divide lettuce onto four plates and place a portion of enchiladas on top. Top with a spoonful of salsa and a dollop of sour cream, tomatoes, and olives.

4 servings

CONCLUSION

We, as Americans, are the fattest nation in the world. There's a reason for that. We eat all of the wrong foods and spend our time in a sedentary lifestyle that allows that food to settle into areas of our bodies where we don't want it to be. That food is then converted into the energy that it was meant to provide, but when we don't use that energy, it turns to fat.

The media doesn't help us either when it comes to a healthy body image. We could be heavier than what our recommended body weight is but still be in great shape. After all, muscle weighs more than fat. But the media has us believe that all women must be a size 4 and all men should be ripped with muscles.

The reality is that body shapes are different and weight should not be our only gauge of how in shape we are. The idea is to be sure we eat healthy and take advantage of the way food is meant to work for us – not against us! When you resolve to take off those extra pounds, your whole mindset has to change in order for you to be successful. You have to change your habits – not only your eating habits, but when you eat and how you eat. As we've shown you, you can eat many foods while trying to lose weight and you don't have to starve yourself in the process. There's nothing you really have to sacrifice, you just have to change a little.

Instead of having flour tortillas, have wheat ones. Instead of eating 5 cookies, just eat 1. Switch to low-fat or no-fat versions of your favorite foods like cheese and sour cream and decrease your portion size to make sure you don't overeat.

Dieting to lose weight doesn't have to be painful or uncomfortable. It can be fulfilling and satisfying and even tasty!

Angela Turner

Now that you have the tools you need, you can modify any of the recipes we've given you and create your very own foods with the "allowed" ingredients. It's up to you to succeed. We know you can! So here's to your slimmer body, but most of all – a healthier YOU!

REFERENCES

The following websites were referenced in researching this book:

www.newcreations.net

www.bodybuildingforyou.org

www.mayoclinic.com

www.bodyforlife.com.

ABOUT THE AUTHOR

I'm very passionate about keeping fit, losing weight, and being well. If I gain even just a few pounds let's say within 2 or 3 months, that means I am not sticking to my workout plan or I am not eating within the guidelines that I write about. And mentally, if I find that things are off in some way, I know it's time for me to get centered again and get my focus back. But I don't make it a major problem. I simply recall the basics of what I know that I should be doing and then in a short while, I'm there again at my goal.

I know this happens to a lot of people, so that's why I try to break things down as reasonably and practical as I can so that anyone can follow and reach any goal that they've set for themselves. It's not easy because we all get sidetracked by different things in life. But I know it's still achievable for me and for you. I'm still going through my journey but with keeping fit and being well, it makes the experience so much better.

www.ingramcontent.com/pod-product-compliance
Lightning Source LLC
Chambersburg PA
CBHW072012290526
45787CB00013B/884